SONNETS

Infected Life, Gifted Breath, Death's Defiance

Robert Witkow

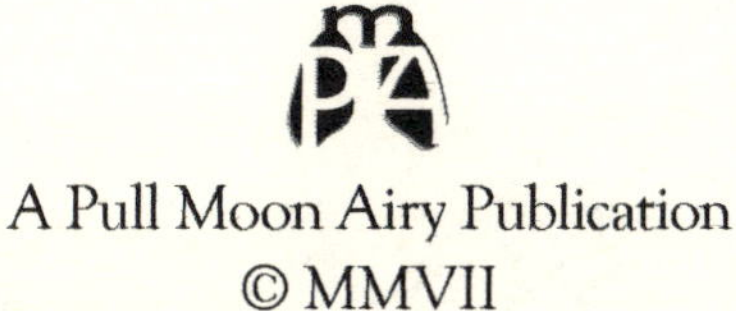

A Pull Moon Airy Publication

Pull Moon Airy Publishing
245 East 63rd Street, Suite 221
New York, NY 10021

www.pullmoonairy.com

ISBN-13: 978-0-615-13775-9
ISBN-10: 0-615-13775-X

Design by David Pitagorsky

First Edition
2007 by Pull Moon Airy Publishing

It is the number one genetic killer of children and young adults in the United States. It cripples airways, swindles breath, inflicts sorrow, condones agony. To my ears, any reference imposed on its behalf mindfully scars, the vaguest of utterances touting its name ensuring subversion. If even soughed in a soliloquy, an incurring wrath descends. When consequence pervades my thoughts, seeds of logic unravel in the preciousness of an instant.

In the early seventies, when a victimized infant was first diagnosed, Hippocratic Oaths were perjured, for some physicians' suggestive means curried an abandonment of hope, disposal of a future. And in the piddling scope of their eyes, to stage instinctive warfare, viably pursue any course of treatment, nurture, as does parental love inherently dictate, was stoutly deemed futile, since impending Death was a statistical certainty. But just as they served to be insolent stooges disgracing their profession, select colleagues, unabashedly diametrical, quintessential to medicine, to the world entire, aspired to impugn such beliefs, to prompt a renaissance both challenging and countering claimed perceptions; driven they were by a striking ambition to eventually impede, contain, and derail its ferocity. Propagate a life desirable as opposed to one despicable.

Yeah, it was true, the numbers didn't lie. But neither did glimmers of infinite prospects, of disregarding projected prognoses, of courting possibilities nestled in the pendulous richness of dreams, the tenuous ticks of Time. Today, all those strains of promise, all disdain for the assumptive, all those beaconed rays of light have become a most miraculous actuality.

These sonnets, a bestowal of devotion, are dedicated to those who have valiantly lost their lives, those endlessly engaged in the fight to persevere, and those who have been afforded the gift of a transplant. A blessèd opportunity to victoriously endure. It is the most selfless of acts to be an organ donor, an astonishing feat of humanity, one of incredible eminence. Tears abound, shed with painful joy in the wake of despair. It is so hard to gain from someone else's loss. Every single breath is a reminder of that.

This disease, cystic fibrosis, it *can* be beaten. I know, because that infant given no chance of survival some thirty-five years ago, was me.

How to pen such an endearing thank you, an ode so resplendent, so profoundly impassioned with admiration's homage, that the words themselves paint a staggering portrait of friendships so gratuitous, so inspirited, that never has there been, nor ever shall there be, kindred prose composed of worthier comparison. But in truth absolute, any attempt to scribe the like would only be evidenced as an ignoble, farcical injustice, for no union of letters, no matter how strung together, could convey such an ever-elusive, ever desirous testimonial. But still, must not I try? To you all, unintentionally caught in the web of my plight, drenched by recurring, unrepentant rainfalls of inconvenience, who, despite my being incapable of reciprocation, showcased an irrevocable love, extending to me, with seemingly effortless exertion, showers of light in the darkest of life's waning hours—just know that held within my aforesaid ramblings, O, how so dutifully I tried.

My parents, who by way of their own forfeiture, have bestowed upon me, with a towering dignity, cascades of tireless, exceptional positivity. A most genuine testament to love, within which adversity was slayed, hope was salvaged, and all the while that doorway to a future was kept gilded and ajar with a will and a prowess that's simply remarkable. How ever such strength, such resolve found their way into your hearts, well, I believe it an impossibility to fathom, for my own rationale decrees decades of a blatant, burdensome existence on my behalf. But it serves as a handsomely guised crutch, self-surveyance carting self-subjugation, fragility condensed over fragments of Time. There is a litany of names, an endless parade of faces that have played differing roles to mend my torn and frayed body throughout the sway of my lifetime. Some have stayed, their visages indelible, their eyes forever swathed with a telling kindness; others have merely faded, blended in as do transitions of reckoning, for no other reason than Time and circumstance. But even still, with respect to the former, we are thrust into each other's realm solely when illness governs it be so. Ah, 'tis you, only you, who always have been there for me, tending to my malaise, infusing me with reassurances, with the perpetuating insistence that tomorrow may hold more promise than does today.

Two pillars that never topple. Medicines, doctors and procedures may have saved my life, but without you, there would have been no life to save.

Dr. Celia Ores, thirty-five years and counting of unwavering regard, uncompromising diligence, relentless commitment. Your brilliant mind habitually reclaims me from the depths of myself, in every way imaginable. With a momentous salience, fears were abated, denials were absorbed; drafts of seasoned truths, of necessitated realisms judiciously fell upon my ears, inflecting an eventual absolution. When episodically careening into morbidity's abyss, swept up in engorging paradigms of downward spirals, you lifted such banes, the number of times incalculable. The impact of having crossed into your threshold, as do my traipsing fingers alone so meritoriously confirm, still leaves me breathless with awe as I ride on breezes fueled by billowy gusts of breath. A rare and precious gem, whose sparkle never dulls, whose worth no value could exceed. Wrapped about my heart shall always be thy convalescing ribbon, specially bowed and forever beknotted with love.

Dr. Brian Scully, ingenious apothecary, dispenser of life-sustaining elixirs. Your demeanor, so even-keeled, your faith, so admirable. Whenever incident finds me in your company, irrespective of reason, a rehabilitative smile is always your escort, a shadow of stability ever your accompaniment. Alas, when breath's desertion was hovering with tactility, and Death's agents were circling about, I awoke to the hallowed vision of you kneeling at my bedside, hands clasped in prayer. To The Virgin Mary you prayed, prayed for a miracle, for a pair of lungs to save a life, my life. And no more than some three hours later, a triteness of insignificance to most, a devouring fury of whisking potency to me, that prayer was answered. And O, doubt I not it was your power of divinity. As much as a savior as She is to you, you are to me. A kinder, sweeter man, graced with a richness of forethought, of faculty, few will ever meet. How blessed I am to be among those few.

Dr. Larry Schulman, harbinger of wisdom, a noble and righteous character. Your temperament beams with contagious grandeur, your humor is slated to unfailingly mend. The poignancy of your understanding instills a restorative blend of confidence and charisma.

Between us there lies a most uncanny connection, an alliance of appreciation that is sure to carry us whimsically, sagaciously onward. We go back a long way, a road paved with captivating travails and cemented with an easeful fondness. Drawn I have always been to anyone whom administers harmonious vibes without motive. And that, though being just a fractional gauge of your embodiment, is a categorical reflection of your wholeness.

Dr. Joshua Sonett, draped in swells of assuagement, a masterful engineer employing an auspicious, salutary finesse of proportions duly insurmountable. That moment when I first did make your acquaintance tarries with the permanence of a tattoo, sparking a fantastical reminiscence, like some fancied reverie so vividly retrievable. It remains prosperously embedded in my psyche with a tangible, spiritual clarity. It was as if Fate, at long last, had delivered to me a flourishing destiny. Wild bouts of trepidation turned to calm, debilitating anxieties to relief. Your surname alone surpassed blind coincidence; quite astounding, really. This sonneteer, though having been enfeebled, summoned introspection; my wits, though detracted, cradled discernment. With a poet's cavalier intuitiveness, my quill, readily dipped to immortalize, to pen the greatest Sonett yet writ, laid forth the foundation of a canonization by plume, whereby invoking boundless gasps of awe by all whom imbibe its puissance, whom feast on its splendor. In you resides a light that preciously glows, that rescues and rekindles with both a medicinal and personal glory. You are a special incarnation of magical persuasion to all whom canvass your masterpieces. How fortuitous I am to consider both yours and Nancy's friendship as one stitched with an inseverable thread.

Peter, Cindy, Jackson and Elizabeth—what a wonderful family; wisdom abundant, strength propitious, support unyielding.

Marjorie and Sam, Janis and Kylie, Caroline, Marc, Gabrielle and Brett—so fortunate to be embraced by you all, though more fortunate still to embrace you back.

My dear, darling friends, age indiscriminate—a cooler bunch of cats I couldn't imagine. As I rapaciously ride down the highway of life, O, perennially saddled up alongside be thy spectred caravan, galloping in

a synchronous, sequenced processional which intrinsically suspends all of adversity's onslaughts. And to unscramble the mysticism, the enigmatic origin of such an occurrence, stands to be as precise as it is ambiguous, as I happened upon its explanative dictation while under the auspices of fatigue, nodding off in the bleakest hours of morn, just as darkness was preparing to give way to the light. O, how it came to be that I secured unfettered pools of beauty from camaraderie's reservoir, from Fortune's reserve, a Camelot from whenceforth our crossroads majestically intersect–must be that 'tis in accordance with Fate's volition. And being as such, I am invariably, tearfully, rendered a speechless cat, a solemn cat, the luckiest cat of all.

David Pit–without you, my friend, this book of sonnets would still remain an unfinished vision. Your time always avails, your talents no less than extraordinary, your tenacity and desire to have brought this to fruition, with an artistry and a perfection, complements and parallels that same glint of pride and purpose mirroring my own. It is as much a reward welcoming its finality as it was throughout every turn comprising the enactment of its creation.

Steadfast custodians of restorative well-being, of reprieves conferred and equally received–from the E.R. to the O.R., surgeons to interns, nurses to aids, coordinators to secretaries, technicians to transporters, house calls to holistic healers, in every city, every country roved, where every realizable, every conceivable aspect of care was afforded my way, I am deeply, distinguishedly indebted.

To that child, now in Heaven, whom Death took too soon, whose breath I now breathe, whose path I now travel–it is difficult for me to express what emotions overtake my musings, the complexities that detail my decipherment of justification and accountability. Churning with constancy so goes the daily crescendos expending my gratitudes, my apologies; and when that day arrives, bringing with it my exodus into sanctuary, into the privileged company of your presence, I know just what shall be conveyed, just what the exacting benefaction my words shall relay. It is my greatest of hopes that during my ephemeral tenure on earth, I am able to reward you in some manner appropriate, some capacity you are excessively deserving of. Stands the very same for that of your family. It is in me that your spirit survives, ever fusing with that of my own, and ever beguiling with breathtaking might.

Tara—

My Love, My Angel, My Muse

One needn't be plucked from the parables of Olympus, be sanctified in a psalm, or be deified in lore to be fitted with wings and a halo. You just hide yours so well.

When the rankest of stenches, the rottenest of visions embroiled my sanity, you cleansed what sludge dragged me down with caresses of permeative love. When fits of revolting coughs hoarded reactionary stares rife with disgust, you ignored such enmity, guiding me to refuge until, by a dual, practiced suppression, respite set in. You are in possession of a patience the strictures of mortality regard as untenable, a beauty I thought only to have existed in verses inked by Keats, a love everblooming, my heart enwreathing, my soul corralling. And so it was, following each Time anew that intravenous dripped its last drop, coursing pathetically through the quixotic instability of my veins, ever and always by my side you were, ready to appease my pressing want to travel the world, from one week jaunts to holy pilgrimages, knowing full well my lungs were slated to fail me, so predictably, so incorrigibly, far too quickly. O, how tragically often and implosively damning was the case, surfacing with a repetition implacable. Yet not once, during all those serialized repugnancies that turned you nursemaid, those sweetest of outings having mutated into souring solitudes, all treks embarked upon turned to bedridden stints, when your own happiness was a sacrificed inevitability, not one time flashed you persuasions tagged with resentment, not ever did a single complaint befall my ears, beget frustration, begrudge your thoughts. And, my love, all those days within months within years I spent withering, wasting away in a hospital bed, so it was you subjecting yourself to that very same; for did nary a night laced with fright come to pass, or a dawn dressed in dismay arrive whereby went absent thy breadth, thy balance, thy consecrated solace, O, so unequivocally enclasped about mine. Were never you granted a break from my misfortunes, which only swept you further into misfortune's bane.

O, how so immeasurably sorry I am, having robbed you of the delicate impulsions, the fugitive dalliances, the serendipitous phenomena Time irretrievably grants within the scope of a decade. Ten years gone, usurped and ransacked, swallowed and lost. The aftermath an immersion of biding self-reflection, the begemming emerald splash of your eyes a passageway into remembrances, into rueful impressionisms of failure and abandonment. Blistering scars of plaintive despondence. But love, as is ours—grippingly pastoral—was borne of a Fate otherworldly. And of such a love, poets romanticize, philosophers hypothesize, dreamers, they fantasize, and writers, well, they can do nothing but plagiarize. Dante and Beatrice. Tristan and Isolde. Romeo and Juliet. Troilus and Cressida. Paris and Helen. Robert and Tara. Hark!—yea, as sure as 'tis truth aft the morn comes the morrow, so too be it a rightful claim, semantically professed, that neither do thine eyes deceive thee nor doth my conjecture miscolor me! O, be it not of ill-mannered propriety to take it upon myself posturing thy rejoinder; declare me a fool!—implicate my pretension as unquantified dribble!—regard my contention as nothing more than a precarious foray into pomposity, into blatant egoism, a provisional gander projecting love buttressed by incursive insecurities! Ah, 'tis indeed not of the mind's invention that the rostered names preceding our own have incontestably, most undeniably set a precedent as to the conceptualized fixity of love's spectra, as corroborated in legend and presided over by the impartiality of Time. But O, never shall I concede that our paradisal footing stands unworthy of inclusion alongside the aforementioned couplets, and that the Heavens shall one day lay home to our eponymous constellation of the brightest order. And O, 'tis just ever so sad chanced these lovers never to have met the likes of us, nor we them, liberated from the constricts of literature.

Our breaths together nurture illumination, embrace transcendence, endure dissension. It is, and continues to be, you whom I hang onto. So much the better than just hanging on to yourself.

O, my dear, sweet angel—this book of sonnets has been penned with that same passion you have suffused my every essence with. It is marked with love, a love unbound, a love eterne.

There have been so many advancements, but still no cure. Yet you, with the purchase of this book of sonnets, have helped further realize that which is our dream, as a portion of the proceeds are being donated to charities dedicated to funding the research that will ultimately bring, to those in need, the beauteous breath of life.

I

Let love as I knew her come once again–
Find me amidst what's been lost by my heart!
I shudder to feel the ill-fates of men
That long have endured love's play with no part;
Now, bleak and torn, by self-imposed duty
Seek I harpèd plucks, thy sweet, am'rous strings,
Whenso play'd, th'Angels, struck by such beauty
Didst fit you to wear most beauteous wings!
Relentless are fires unleashed to belie;
O, desertion nears, all of hope subverts!
Agonized throes acquaint tears to mine eye,
Carved of betrayal, guised cravèd desserts;
   To love all thy days, the nights would I tame–
   Felled blind or fed sight, my love binds selfsame!

II

By light of the morn I quiver with fear,
Knowing but not if this soul shall suspire;
Jaded by visions profoundly austere,
The breadth of unknown consumes me entire.
Shadows besiege the meridian hour;
No tarot, nor sibyl, nor diviner's chart
Didst trag'dy read; O, dread forgèd Fate sour!–
Dear bane of existence, chance you depart?
Brusque fall of day uproots downtrodden blight,
Ushering in all that madness befriends;
Flick'ring, Death's candles burn wicked with sleight–
Alit at sun's rise, snuff'd whence daylight ends.
As darkness decrees, Time hath light swindled;
No creat're mayst snatch breathèd breaths Time's dwindled.

III

O, purlèd whispers from soft lips assuage
Such rueful throbs of this lonesome dreamer;
Breaths eagerly drawn insatiably engage
This heart to uphold no love supremer!
Resurrection, aged five, hast requiem's
Mass silenced!–Immaculate Conception
Didst fearlessly seal my mausoleum's
Gateway, hence precluding Death's reception!
O, birthright wrongèd hath reap'd Labors Twelve;
"With Herculean might," quoth I, "shed blood
To pain's scheme impede dreamt of depths love'll delve;"
Truth marks my mettle, cometh fire or flood!
Dreams o'er-sway dreams, yet e'er-fixed dreams of you
Possesseth my fancies dreamt hereunto.

IV

As sure as sleep's realm resplendently streams
Spectral blasts of electrified folly,
Beauty exquisite m'lady embeams
So as to purge ingrain'd melancholy.
Infatuation enraptures thy lure–
Passion emblazon'd most undeniable;
Revered satisfaction prevails to cure–
Laudation whelm'd most justifiable.
Phidias, his Athena, amazeth
E'en th'artless: veiled gold, ven'rable iv'ry–
Yet stand thee beside, all eyes shift to gazeth
'Pon beauty the likes Grecians ne'er 'll 'gain see!
  As doth disease siphon reason from poem,
  My lov'th chimeric recedes with each gloam!

V

The night ere last sallow moon shed Her sheath,
Rising in nakedness, smiling deceit;
'Fore didst affection's dew e'er douse Her wreath,
She fled from the sky in hasty retreat.
Celestial huntress's stellar domain–
The trail of Her wake with ambiv'lence teems;–
Hazèd by dustings blush'd faint be'st star's reign:
Subject and setting of fairy tale themes;
Ah, Fate intervened!–their sov'reigns, undone,
Their crowning, gleam'd splendor now forsook cold!
Whimsical folklore whisks parody's pun;
Storybook endings be'st storied lies told!–
If yarns, spun to hear, ope'd 'once 'pon a time',
Read never wouldst I 'the end' of penned rhyme.

VI

Glancing thy way, I could not deny love,
Or love, dare I say, would not deny me;
This heart hath been seized, left thriving thereof,
Bespellèd by Freyja's ain vanity!
Tidal woes (maelstroms of hysteria)
Ægir's seas devise; Odin well abides
As down dives His maiden Valkyria–
To Valhalla's Feast of Heroes She rides!
Loki's contrivers of discord defend
Thor's rattling thunders, served to e'er bludgeon
All mine app'tencies! O, ne'er I intend
Abeyance, behoove to act Gods' gudgeon!
O dear, kind'st Freyja, please quencheth my thirst,
For of love, I fear, this soul hath been cursed!

VII

Erenow I dreamt 'pon a storm-ridden night
My love, forged distinct, gone 'midst the thunder;
A grave, dug shallow, requests by invite
One-way passage wher'st Death swirls asunder!
Whom else couldst ruse jasper eyes, sprinked gold dust?–
Cumber my breath, footholds further denied?–
Turn swellèd lips, swathed cerise, stung robust,
To torturous percepts swept unespied?
Just one kiss be all, one taste of love's spice;–
Who'd then prove skilled to disjoint one from the
Other? E'en eterne, prom'sing pleas, pled thrice,
Couldn't entice this dream to deserteth me!
  The world, 'twas well-shoulder'd on Atlas's strength–
  Lik'ned burd'n I'd bear to encase thy love's length!

VIII

Brisk affair, love-led, soughed brash at my door;
Bereft, inside she stepped, a sinning saint
Whose act was quaint and dainty to the core.
Snow-blinding flakes (as yet thawed) felled me faint,
Massing abundant, my heart o'erpow'ring;
Feigned supplications claiming subversion
Answerèd were via vestal white show'ring–
Ashore, 'pon tides, ensures she coercion!
From stern to bow, O, she's glazèd in rime–
Glacial libations drench'd of hypnotism;
If love were to blind, toward blindness I'd climb,
Swathe crystalline eyes love's visional prism!
For reasons unknown, know need'st I thy niche
Wher'st grips of cold churn out love's warmth so rich.

IX

Purposed by will, seek I love's lightning strike;
Pure glow, resilient to Nyx, shines o'erhead
Mine angel: Gods, mortals be'st lured alike
T'eye such beauty eyes ne'er 'fore hath eyèd!
If chanc'd I thy love t'immeas'rably hold,
All of life's riches couldn't enrich love's mirth,
For po'try's tongue shall wile Wit into gold;
Spurn'd!–scant wealth, coin'd Ploutus, love can't outworth!
O, jailed;–charg'd, shamm'd passion! Welcome, Hell's mire!
Magistrate's jurists: stooged fools, truths decoyed;–
Sentenc'd to life lovelorn! Grief sets my pyre,
Fashion'd as Dido's aft Aeneas's void!
The heavens, so swell'd, impart gilded wings,
Repairing their loss whilst gain I suff'rings!

X

A festered dolor hath airèd this morn,
Slithered o'er Time with reptilian's lurk;
Dealt nary an ally, stand I so lorn–
Prey sacrificial 'midst Death's fixèd smirk.
Vices invective beget ill-gotten
Penance, visèd by tyrannical clutch;
Poison, slow-released, wears my veins rotten–
O! rippeth me from vile, vulturous crutch!
A brewing vendetta emboils untamed,
Rabid for vengeance, for gorgèd bloodshed;
Flaunt breath as bait?–Fool!–My soul'll ne'er go claimed
By thee, leech! Life's lust shant be pirated!
Skulking in shrouds abets thy vehicles,
Fueled to attain the direst pinnacles.

XI

O, long hath canny Time harbor'd Her guise–
Vapid displays dous'd replete with self-love;
Watch'd She: Paradise Lost, Devils uprise
To 'gainst God rebel, thence Man Regain love!
With prowess, She sways what biddings await–
Lain forth for I be unfulfill'd morrows!
Her dupe, 'twas Eden 'fore Satan hung bait–
Evil's Tree leaves No Ledge, just ring'd sorrows!
Be sooth'd by Her chimes, but be not seduced–
By pact drawn with Death, dual evils conspire;
Amused best they be whence breaths be reduced
To paltry attempts to barely respire;
The clarion call of Death's lurid howls
Echoes in shadows wher'st infamy prowls.

XII

Do whet this lovelorn fool so deficient
Of that which compels the heart to flutter;
Infuse me with thy counsel omniscient–
Bathèd desires purported to shudder!
Bestow upon my nature laconic
Sprightly swells of almighty emotion;
Teach to me of said feelings symphonic–
Do exorcise love's raging demotion!
Breathlessness nears–hear'st not Donne's bells tolling?
Hark! sweet silence sings! O, 'tis for I whom
Death's knells, Devotions tell, ceased their knolling!
Perchance, be it true, love's bane shant resume?
What powers thee hold, all Magi lay awed;
Thy magic beheld, my heart doth belaud!

XIV

On A Gift Of Five And Twelfth

Whenso angels egress their heav'nly bed
Intent on ascribing wings sewn of gold,
Upon thy doorstep they land, garlanded,
To enthrone unmarred beauty Gods extolled!
No depth of seas, nor widths to take measure,
Nor breath's serenade, nor lengths love forgoes
Fathomably couldst fail to entreasure
The most beaut'ous pose e'er etchèd in prose!
Covetous eyes immersed broad in disgust
O'ertake Aphrodite, o'ercome with disdain,
For Fate did fell Her to opt to entrust
Her beaut'ous reign o'er to thee to ordain!
Golden bright halo now 'bove thee doth shine;
Thy depths, widths, breaths and lengths my dreams'll enshrine!

XV

Choral, infatuate ballads appease,
Their oft-rehears'd melodies mesmeric;
Harmony's chime rides on Time's graceful breeze–
Each hour denoted by knells chimeric.
Kinkèd red ringlets (so lewd) kept me slewed–
Kimono wide ope (thoughts swarm) didst becharm;
Sleek downward slide, undress'd temptress stands nude–
O, curvaceous lust displodes love's alarm!
Rare be'st thy beauty, more so each new light;
"Selene," spurr'd I, "do devour Death's scheme;
Retract not thy beam, stay full long this night–
Hypnos convince life exists chance to dream!"
'Fate doom'd he die young,' so marketh my tomb;
'A bride ne'er he held–O, befell'd, cheat'd groom!'

XVI

Morgan le Fay: crude sorceress by craft,
Incestuous vamp, enchantress depraved;
Conjuring Merlin, his wizardry daft–
Dare them cross, by spells incant'd be'st enslaved!
Wanton diversions, determined to seethe,
Avail'd Guinevere's thrusts promiscuous;
Whence prick'd by Lancelot's sword, lusts unsheathe–
Camelot crumbled; O, knight traitorous!
Love impaled Arthur 'fore ever didst steel–
Mordred's blade, unrepentant undoer!
'Twas Avalon wher'st wound'd King fail'd to heal;
O, well-round'd ruler, whoe'er reign'd truer?
Glory-fill'd legends mayst ever Tales keep,
Tho none, save Chaucer's, cut bawdily so deep.

XVII

Treacherous woe, here again! Breath's sleekest
Mauler, crownèd by kings as Death's crudest!
O, birthèd lame; persecuted, weakest
Runt from lioness's womb! Sacked by shrewdest,
Iniquitous cripplings; grisly, grimmest
Bouts of suffocation breed life's shrillest
Wails! O, repulsiveness prevails! Dimmest
Pitfalls engulf a malaise of illest
Venoms; inherited genes impurest!
Fearful and wearied, bloods coughèd starkest
Serve spoilage of dreams! Cannot endurest,
Raped of purpose! Good riddance, days darkest!
   Confess, I must, thy course be the slyest;
   Thy hand, I'll take, when ride thee the nighest.

XVIII

A hunger impellent again doth call;
Threshèd, Hell-bred, pain-fed lacerations
Demonically, peccantly bemaul!
O, do bedamn breath's exacerbations!
I thirst, desirous, to rid what virus
Capitulates to none, save one, save Death;
Scourged, ghastly cries veraciously pious
Tarry so as my lot ne'er doth tempereth!
"To war," harped Death, "breath I'll annihilate!"
O, robb'd by spite wast Wit's benevolence–
Lungs condemned shalt my hearse facilitate!
O, too ravag'd, too raped by malevolence!
Perhaps horrid darkness offers the light
Through which tired bones need no longer to fight.

XIX

Cursèd spirits, scent of Hell–collective
Shards of discord rain upon my rapture;
Sprung of the inferno, breaths defective
Sadistically seal betimes sepulcher.
Hate's attrition assembles voracious
Pangs raw with destruction; circling about
Be leisure's torment rifling tenacious
Rapports, diabolically doled out.
Perditious toxins molest pulmonic
Strides by means methodically om'nous;
Rancor wallows in rejections chronic–
O, despicable bastard vainglor'ous!
Slink coward, from thy shell; show me power
I deem true, then at my hands you'll cower.

XX

As thy passion enveined sweeps 'neath my skin
(A seduction self-possess'd by treason),
Conquests you flaunt, dastardly paladin–
Unchaste perversions chased with filthed reason.
Can't thee 'mbrace threads stitchèd of sympathies,
Quelleth hate's will with quilts patchèd to mend?
Will'st tear-dress'd, remorse-drench'd soliloquies,
Scenes lined with lies, acts derailed, ever end?
O, canst sick'ning macabre be purgèd?
Is mercy no more than a merc'less dream?
Enfeeblement, health's mirth–O, whence mergèd,
Insuff'rable void besets my regime!
Yea, 'tis but truth I do weep out thy name,
Yet nay be it truth I recoil with shame.

XXI

Of hands life's dealt, hellacious comes to mind;
Stands much the same for banes parasitic.
'Tis on'y but Death whom holds five of a kind–
Anted my soul t'enfolds cataclysmic!
Bound to e'er suffer be'st Time's contrivance,
A deliberate, fiendish dissection;
Strive I to rive Death's angels' survivance–
Undying be'st my pride's insurrection!
By no means shalt thy plagues be forgiven,
By no means shalt thee be my outwitter,
By no means shalt acquittance be given,
By no means shalt thee brand me "submitter".
  Dreams birthed as fancies, reveries fed sweet
  Only toward foulness churn, fueled by deceit.

XXII

O merciless Time, have mercy on me–
I am a messenger lost but in love;
Seek out another and leave me to be–
Thy legion elite I'm worthy not of.
Agèd yon oak's listless limbs hang threadbare–
How chance he to smile left nary a leaf?
And there, to the west, that thrice-wounded mare–
Shall not she give thanks allayed of such grief?
O merciless Time, delay my demise–
Indeed there are nobler souls to be had;
Tho waif-like and meek, my strength in love lies–
O merciful Time, do o'erlook this lad!
Been spared, lest for now, but e'er doth Time loom–
Clever pallbearer availing my tomb.

XXIII

Time cues Her dance with each delicate tick,
Advancing visage revising whoms age
Shalt diminish by choreographed snick;
Aristocrat's court, sweet minuet's stage!
Time trills Her song–"Dies Irae" She plays–
Hymned lament rolling of peals, trolling raps;
O, fancy She does Her voice duly sways
Pearled baroque organ to pipe my collapse!
Time seeks Her prey with practiced precision,
Glancing with glazed, abominable smile;
With scythe to lead She rives Her incision,
Striking a deal whereby Fate serves up guile!
Be wary days now, and all that await;
Time's sentence swoops down, dispensing Death's date.

XXIV

The sun, as secured by chariot crossed,
Hath ris'n again, egocentric and vain,
Dowsing the nightfall with schemes to accost
That bastion I bask in to wile the pain.
O, e'en alchemist's potions kissed ill-laced,
Shant, 'pon consumption, summon Death's campaign,
For Love's own footsteps by love'll be retraced
To unfix what Fate's tricks didst foreordain!
Born famished of breath, obituaries
Read: "A life infringed ends on dead end street."
O, alive still to fend!–down on knelt knees
Pray I the sun's beam be deemed obsolete!
Tho night's arrival drops daylight's curtain,
Lead Star's performance anon plays certain.

XXV

"Do what thou wilt shall be th'whole of the Law,"
The Great Beast himself (Crowley) didst proffer
As Aiwass, his Muse, lent tongue to his claw;
O, magick Qabalist, black worshipper!
Delusions invade when eyelids are drawn–
There, reprieve's been mapped, chance flight through a cloud;
O, hope dies! Ruination's ruse, aimed to spawn
Reviling dawns, now airs successes proud!
Trapped in sleep's maze, walled in by zeal's jackals;
O, come blue bird, sing 'scape melodious–
My Theseus be; shatter dream's shackles,
Decry names kin to demons odious!
That realm whereof I drink from love's chalice
Grants me the will to rid of sleep's malice.

XXVI

Only but love now doth keep me alive–
My Tara, her breadth, be all that I long;
Between stolen breaths, what lusts we revive!
"Dear Death, in full-dress, we fear not thy song!"
Whence Hell's air, swept rancid, swarms 'bout the room,
Roses, fresh-plucked, shalt its fester repel;
Whence shadows, opaque, scour light to entomb,
Haloes of joy shalt its Darkness dispel!
A lean, hungry look holds whom wields Death's knife;
O! dual stabs to destroy?–both Love denied!
Prevailed thee wouldst, staked but one heart with strife;
Slay two?–O! too much love hurls Death aside!
    As much as a ripple helps feedeth the sea,
    Amour shall bind our love infinitely.

XXVII

I say, fair kingdom, pluck ye selves from fields
Filled of poppy, give tired hands a furlough
From toil! Come gather, dear friends, the breeze yields
Such bellows! O, what Joy! all is aglow!
With festive song, proclaim I 'bout the land
That a frolic of fancy is hereby
Deemed law! Reach for that sweet syrup at hand!
Dance th'estampie engarbed to dandify!
Love's back, I say, back to set hearts afire!
Alabaster wink, slung like strings of pearls,
Gleans grand as diamond snowfalls! Let the lyre
Benumb with roaringly, rapturous swirls!–
Yea verily, Love drums melody's mewl!–
Juggling Love's gestures, this jester's Love's Fool!

XXVIII

Behold the delphinium's wind-swept spikes–
Beauty, by gander, depth'd deadly design;
Coquettish assassin's pistil-whipp'd strikes
Trigger my tendrils whilst sepals entwine;
O, salacious stamen stalks stylized leaves
Swell'd ripe to invite, stigmatically sprawl'd;
Pussy willow's pollen this King Bee thieves,
Plush soil implanting 'fore in gard'n bed crawl'd!
Exotic impulsions, sown O very
Climactic–blooming lusts groom'd to conceive;
Vibration's treat penetrates thy Cherry
Tree's sweet sap, which came didst I to retrieve!
Deflow'ring thy flow'r full-whets my app'tite–
Tulip's ablossom, two lips fed delight!

XXIX

Whence drunk, potion's pretense vowing amour
Subscribes unto notions that advocate
Love; ah! Cupid's hoax, no more! O, abhor
I fallacy's lore, need'st denunciate
Foul'st of claims! Gullèd abidance besmear,
For minds markèd implicitly adept
Best those fed corrupt tidings! All revere
Love's loathers, slight whomst t'love loathe lay inept!
Found I, by chance, which did long dust conceal,
Stealth'ly drawn maps whose engravings exhume
Encoded clues, once deciphered, reveal
Love's incurred wrath 'twill all lovers entomb!
Contrary whims, if right read, Wits expose
Opposing inversions writ verses enclose.

XXX

As Eros approach'd my dark, lonely door,
In shrouds I endur'd, eyes quiv'ring with fear;–
"Make haste, Erida, rouse hatred to gore
Cherub's winsome zeal–slay love's cavalier!"
Archer's device, arrows five dippèd sweet;
Cunning panacea coat'd gold varnish,
Its sheen assured to love absorb, to mete
Out silver'd ploys, thence their purity tarnish!
Daughters of Zeus, artful Muses, entice
Bemusing maneuvers pand'ring romance;
Their passionless state besets Paradise,
Ensuring, at best, abject circumstance!
  A sleuth, well-play'd, eyes what mirrors reflect;
  By Wit, words transposed pose truths indirect.

XXXI

Love hath afforded these eyes to believe
That beauty, in all incarnations known
(Venus's recipes), angels didst thieve–
A robb'ry only couldst Graces condone!
Met thee love's unholiest prophecy?–
The Messiah hast no brethren to bless!
Bishops thence dispel fectious anarchy
By citing temptation's path to excess!
Writ gospels of saints be christened often
Pois'nous, mauling truth with cagey deceit;
Betray'l (pure Judas) coaxes my coffin–
In vain!–light shines, crucifixions retreat!
 Riddle of Sphinx, Oedipus solved by wit;
 Dark rites of Death's shroud did Wit's light decrypt.

XXXII

If love transcendent be cause to indict,
Then this soul do convict, birth namèd Wit;
Provideth my quill a means to indite;
Papyrus or bark, care I not a whit,
For tho edicts ban love, my voice, my word
Shall right submit true to lawed ordinance,
To papal canons (plaintively pained, whirred
Bluff of Men's Rights). Thence, love's ink wilt ordnance
Assume, arm'd parchment firing illusive
Acts detailing a tryst, styled to incite
Escapist escapades, drawn elusive
As flakes of snow–Swiss Guards lack all insight!
Words mayst read absurd, yet whence spok'n aloud
Hum a hymn, hid herein, wittily allowed!

XXXIII

Drub me with perilous taunts of defeat?–
Pitiful Siren, what course hast thee drawn?
Pull away, turn thy wings, hamper thy fleet–
How hath such wickedness made you its pawn?
Sonorous verse's sole intent–maraud
This mariner faring blustery swells;
I seek but a home, a bastion abroad
Whilst thy songed decoys cast enchanting spells!
Chasten thy chords that summon destruction;
Taketh flight, retreat to thine isle of crags–
Ah! wax-fill'd ears defy lured seduction!–
Onward, fair seamen,–hoist victory's flags!
The sea is becalmed, a wreckage forestalled;
Swift now we sail ere we're fore'er enthralled!

XXXIV

When fire, immortal, Prometheus stole,
Zeus curried vengeance, apparent thereof;
Unbound fury ensued, harped wast Death's toll–
Taloned prey, onslaught's eyes, circled above!
Now, I too forebode myth's dooming sequel–
Swift retribution for act deemed taboo;
My crime?–needled blasphemy sans equal;–
Aphrodite's name inked lewd in tattoo!
O! consequence thus strikes subsequent blows,
Rousing from slumber that God amongst Gods;
A bed, lava-lain, beneath me now flows–
Charon, coin-bribed, ferries fav'rable odds!
Through fiery Hell 'pon Styx's savage tide
Scheming I veer, primed to leave Zeus green-eyed!

XXXV

Platonic remotion–monogamous
Exile of mindful, screened masturbation;
Angular slants–jilted, androgynous
Strains of contaminant's molestation.
Maligning misanthropes drone morosely–
Caustic, prejudicial evangelists
Promoting fallacious points verbosely;
Factions cloned furthest from romanticists.
Sexuality explored shiftily,
Lascivious reveries begotten,
Effectual love driven thriftily;
Muses quixotic swiftly forgotten.
Erotic, sadistic acts dramatized;
Erratic delusions thus sonnetized.

XXXVI

As lilies burgeon 'pon boughs blossomed grand,
Just when morn's dew sparkles so dignified,
Flown feathered-bright bird rests her wings to land;
Slipped through Hera's Gate, her perch my bedside!
Sweet blue jay, my thoughts replay thy song's trills
Whose refrains melodic sustain me still;
Honey-dress'd tea, nipp'd with rye, heal'd my ills—
O, why Eva, why bowed thee to Death's will?
Nested in truth, loss finds realism's sigh–
O, once brilliant blues now drift cloud'd in grays;
Dreams lent us Time–home to Max, off you fly;–
O, mem'ries emboss the doldrums of days!–
Hark! thy grand sun's gloom-stain'd, dismal with bale;–
Each waning moon waxes dimm'd shades of pale.

XXXVII

"Dear friend of denial, do silence my squalls
And set to repair my heart's gaping hole;
Hostile, Grim's trespass scaled lionized walls–
Leo's roar, silenced!" O, well met was Death's goal!
What great poems read we: blithe Keats, Kilmer's psalm;
'Midst Great Wars bridged he peaced roads to Lucerne;
Woe! in vile Crab crawled, ten-armed shell t'embalm!
By God's tree rests he now, 'neath Beauty's urn.
Off once drew dawn, swept in sleep, wept I sound–
Gilded, grey mane framed sallow complexion;
Fanciful soul hath Fate mightily crowned–
Spilt teardrops resound laughter's inflection;
Thy song lay so envi'd, with angels you've flown;
Grieved Ceil yarned a deal–now shares she thy throne.

XXXVIII

When woeful whims infuse me with rancor,
Ropèd eyes be by lanyard beleaguered;
"Zephyrus," I conjure, "hoist moor'd anchor.
Old Salt, mind the masts–fasts left me meagred!"
Death docks abreast; breath deteriorates,
Thrashèd by tides, disabl'd by seaside wheeze;
Undertow wretchedly obliterates,
Submerging 'fore surging rancid disease.
Be'st when savage grief, so rigid and cruel,
Capsizes calm, repels healing weather,
I summon what means to Death overrule–
Tho sunk'n, e'er salvag'd from regions nether!
My love, 'tis you who doth make me believe
Adrift or if drown'd, brine's rogues couldn't love thieve.

XXXIX

'Fore I did breathe blessèd breaths I now own,
Brought on by mandates genetics couldn't mease,
"Mother Mary," pray'd Scully, "chaperon
Lungs; save one of God's children, save him, please!"
O, heard didst She, as my miracle came,
But too came great sorrow; though sav'd one life
Was, one Death overcame. O, youthful flame,
Vivid shines Heaven–thy glow rem'died strife!
Grace! a lung'd trance plant'd itself in the light–
Sweet, treasured chest full of untainted air,
So bountiful, so beautifully bright!–
My only hope be'st my savior's aware;
Breathe I gift'd breaths, as too soon Death you met–
How ever doth one repay such a debt?

XL

To Shakespeare
Upon Reflection Of His Death

What brand of magic bespellèd thy quill,
Elegance bathèd by eloquent plume?
Whose will willed it so that great beauty will
Seep from thy parchment to parch love-swept gloom?
From whence come such words that whisk away loss,
Then argue to gain lost hopes next refrain?
How doth a sadness, so sweeping and cross,
Give way to gladness in scripts ye have lain?
Who cannot sample how tenderness tastes,
Or bathe in a breath that Tyche hath blown,
Or grab sun-drenched rays full-dressed in sweet bastes
Had not thee scribed scenes etched worthy in stone?
Love's feverish aches speared holes in my heart,
Willed by thy name, Bill well hid, billed love's art.

XLI

When scowl and scorn breed a madness unkind,
Burrowing blithesome to bury remorse,
Fears that enrage stage aggressions that bind,
Propell'd to disparage love's baited course.
I held her, but once, her hand soft in mine;–
In swept affliction, and grimness next came,
Cloak'd in a blackness of dreadful design
No tongue dare whisper the wretch of His name!
O, what beauty bore she, like none before–
Locks ringlet red matchèd lips lacquer'd gold;
Alack! lilies, dress'd white, her carriage wore–
O, poor child's life churn'd sour; Death turn'd her cold!
Blind me, as such be a hand by a glove,
Still in dreams will'st I find her, guid'd by love!

XLII

To Father

A king am I, aristocrat by birth;
My father, anointed, a preceptor
To his realm, caprine who knew not a dearth
Of courage, bequeath'd to me a scepter,
An heraldic truncheon steep'd in battles,
Burnt of heroes vanquish'd, their chivalry
Embedd'd in swell'd crests sounding death rattles–
Chronicled sagas charg'd with gallantry!
And now, his hand doth guide my dominion;
A pundit, a prophet bath'd in justice,
And by all accounts, all fair opinion,
A man whose kingship knew no artifice.
Unlike Icarus, life's labyrinth 'scaped I–
'Twas thee, my Daedalus, the reason why.

XLIII
To Mother

'Pon fableist fare, Euterpe my guide
(Hesperides lea to Poseidon's seas),
None shall achieve to e'er stagger my ride–
O! gloweth this Son as the great Pleiades!
Valiantly hued, lit eterne, ne'er to fade,
Mother Sun's divine breath doth nourisheth
Innate, her lullaby's sweet serenade
Eases malaise Death's lurch shant severeth!
Birth's chords; love tied incomprehensible–
O, quintessential, bright angel of earth!
E'er my nurturer indispensable–
O, August's child of bestyled, untold worth!
Sung praise Muses Nine, thine own sonneteers!
Cry out Graces Three–five and fifty more years!

XLIV

In all the lands whenceforth beauty abounds,
'Tis but here, 'pon these fair and dainty shores,
Whereby the sweetness of thy name resounds
By way of the nightingale's fiery scores.
Sated with fuchsias of cinnamon casts,
Thy lum'nous garden illuminates breadth,
Beckoning morrows to summon the pasts
When seeds of dissension first were fedeth.
And I, my love, lay driven to thy lair,
Suffused with desires igniting allure;
No rose grows as beaut'ous, nor couldst one e'er–
Behold! such love incites love's lit'rature!
  O, beauty may rove all about this sphere,
  But none hath more beauty than you, my dear!

XLV

Love me but not for the glory to love,
Nor share in my grief with hopes of esteem,
Nor shelter my hand as such doth a glove
Only to rein pity gamèd to scheme;
Quiet my screams not to trumpet thy drone,
Nor feign burden's wrath in acts dramatized,
Nor sponge up these tears to wring out thine own
Presuming acclaim in hymns eulogized;
Supplicate not for assuagement of pain
Solely to extricate personal woe,
Nor slip from thy lips an air of disdain
When frailty of breath thy Fate shall forgo;
O, down Tara swoon'd,–mine angel was sent!–
A gift of the Gods of no equiv'lent!

XLVI

Matters not Time, nor place, nor occasion,
For this heart shalt ne'er dissever from thine;
'Tis but with love I bide thy invasion–
Ascendancy wheel'd by astral design.
Paint, as though deified, doused my brushes,
Canvassing colors of Fate's conception;
Transportive eyes, they stimulate rushes–
Smile ethereal fractures perception!
Oil-swathed waters balk all navigation–
Swashbuckling pigments, by mutiny, stole
Divine light to embloom my salvation;
With Muse astride, I shall e'er go the vole!
Eternal I am by a love so sound–
Mine angel and me, a portrait unbound!

XLVII

Behold'n in awe be whome'er eyes thy jewel–
A gem laced entire of plumb elegance;
Envy herself became envy's own fool–
Narcissus, 'twas writ, didst shed arrogance!
Bequeath, if thy will'st, the will to suppose
Full-fountain'd leas, o'ergrown orgies of wine;
Bacchus, besotted, to thee didst propose,
"Thy lips,–one swill,–vineyards lush all be thine!"
Benumb'd lashes blinks be enslaved to cease;
Apollo's gilt Temples, drubb'd by thy light!
Eos, enamored, bade you waken Greece;
Hesperus ceded–thee escort the night!
Olympus to Delphi teem'd with delight;
"Tara," Zeus term'd, "be the tenth Muse forthright!"

XLVIII

Beauty's triumvirate flawless doth burn:
In cantos divine didst Dante recall;
Obsessed, 'twas thy kiss Rodin carved eterne;
Mozart's sonatas didst e'er thee enthrall!
Love's couplet rivets in worths yet denied:
Mad went Van Gogh whence thine absence didst come;
Blank canvas so pain'd! Keats, breathless bedside,
Will'd thee an ode 'fore to Death didst succumb!
Purity's longing frames one-line refrain:
Weep! Shelley's Adonais, sweet elegy,
Shines on; O, love 'twill e'er lordly remain,
E'en aft life's Swan Song ushers infancy!
Blest by infin'ty with beauty so rare,
Muse, Grace or Goddess to thee can't compare.

XLIX

When, in all my days of sullen demise,
I ponder Death's truth, if love too shall die,
If agony's daze shalt days agonize
And tears, lonely born, are all tears I'll cry;
O, impish sprite, be they dreams spun by loom?
A tap'stry blooming 'fore love hath begun?
Eyes splashèd em'rald my heart doth consume–
Such beauty beheld be behold'n by one!
By wit, kowtow I; my prayer's sole desire–
Turn passion's spark into love's raging flame;
O! beauty cometh alive like a fire
That sings of sweet love and Tara's that name!
What joy! artful Eros hath struck my heart
For all Time assuring our love'll ne'er part!

L

Wrought of a fire, my Fate pitted against
Fortune's divide wrung with twisted appeal;
Our window of Time bides seasons condensed
(Shifts incidental); ah! love's constant wheel
Doth persevere! Deterrents vile dissolve
With the advent of thy breath! Warmth beyond
Golden throbs (nectared, ripe bliss) circumvolve
My torso! Love forgone was once I fond
Till whipping winds of prosp'rous composure
Didst shepherd repair, ush'ring allayment
Past unguard'd walls! At last, banned disclosure
Drummed out! O, thoughts abandon betrayment!
Of thee, my love, my voice rings poetic,
Drawn, in awe, to thy beauty magnetic.

LI

To Tara
The Only Love Shall Ever I Know

Thou art more beautiful than roses full bloom,
Than skies in waiting to bury the sun,
Than preening flamingo's masterful plume,
Than rainbows awak'ning in unison.
Thou art more sacred than presence of life,
Than burdens that Christ endured on the Cross,
Than vows spoke by man engaging his wife,
Than knights sworn to bear the Grail's albatross.
Thou art more precious than breaths deeply drawn,
Than miracles births enrapture sublime,
Than promising dreams a new sleep may spawn,
Than all of love's poems writ all throughout Time.
Thou doth possess of all that I cherish;
Thy love lost, by my troth, I shall perish.